Introduction

Is your neuropathy destroying the quality of your life?

1) What are your nerve symptoms? Some of the most common: numbness, burning, tingling in the hands, fingers, toes, or feet
2) Do you feel like you're walking on glass, pebbles, or sponges?
3) Do you get horrible cramping in the calves, legs, or feet?
4) Do these cramps keep you awake at night?
5) How long have you been having these symptoms?
6) Do you get them throughout the whole day?
7) Does it interfere with golf, tennis, walking, exercising, or any other activities that you enjoy?
8) Do you have balance issues?
9) Are you unable to walk or stand for long periods of time?
10) Is the problem progressing from your toes and moving up the legs?
11) Is the problem also occurring in your arms and hands?

These issues make up a broken record of what I hear from patients suffering from neuropathy and other chronic conditions.

Does This Sound Familiar to You?

- You need to LEARN TO LIVE with your neuropathy symptoms!
- Once a nerve dies, there's ABSOLUTELY NOTHING YOU CAN DO to help it!
- Your problem COMES WITH AGE.

And in the end, they DO NOT explain how you can BE PROACTIVE—unless it involves taking one of their medications, *which are actually meant for treating seizure disorders* (Neurontin, Gabapentin, Lyrica).

I promise you that my goal is to walk you down a path so that you can take charge of your own health once and for all and actually achieve the goals that you deserve. You only have one life to live, and you need to live your life to the highest level possible. We deserve to be able to look back at our lives without wondering what life would have been like if things had been different or if we had made different decisions. The classic saying is, "The scariest thing is meeting the person you could have been."

We all live in a medical system where we were raised to believe that there is a pill for everything. The problem with this mentality is that pills treat symptoms, not the problem. I take pride in helping patients take charge of their own health once and for all, giving them the power to increase the quality and quantity of their lives.

On your journey through this book, I will show you how it IS possible to achieve the neuropathy symptom relief results that you're looking for.

Chapter 1: Who Am I?

My name is Dr. Adam Zuckerman, and I've been actively treating patients with peripheral neuropathy since 2003. Through the years, I have discovered my "secret sauce" of how to increase the chances of results with neuropathy symptoms. My approach is unique in many ways, in that I treat the body *as a whole*.

My office treats chronic conditions. I specialize in helping patients who are overmedicated, over-injected, and in many cases, over-surgerized, and who finally want to get off the hamster wheel. They are looking for answers, and I take pride in staying ahead of the curve so that I can provide the best quality of care possible to my patients. My unique perspective focuses on each individual person.

So why do I do what I do? Well, from on an early age, I knew I wanted to work with the human body and help people. I remember, as far back as grade school, that while everyone else was checking out fiction books from the library, I was the one reading up on how our bodies work. The more I read, the more I needed to understand as much as possible, and I was utterly fascinated by the amazing human machine.

The more I learned and I educated myself, the more I couldn't understand why people were so quick to take medications and opt for risky surgeries. It just didn't make sense to me. The human body is amazing. The heart beats on its own. The cells of your body can regenerate to the point that a year from now, you're literally a new person. Food can go into the small intestine, and enzymes from the pancreas know to be released. We breathe without giving it any thought. If you cut your arm, blood will circulate, clot, and then scab over and create new skin within a couple of weeks! Doesn't it seem like medications and surgeries would work *against* that process?

I mean, don't get me wrong—I do believe that there's a time and a place for drugs and surgery. It just doesn't make sense to me that people don't operate with the thought process of exhausting all noninvasive methods FIRST. We live in a system where we have all been taught to think of health from an outside-in perspective, forgetting that we were born with the amazing ability to heal.

Society has actually normalized the thought process of symptom-relief pill-popping, wherein you have a common symptom, and without even a thought, you run for the drug that you remember seeing on TV to help resolve the symptom. You never give even one thought to treating the cause, let alone looking into what actually led to the symptom. It's like seeing your vehicle's check engine light come on and putting a piece of duct tape over it. You may have covered up the symptom, but the underlying problem will lead to your engine frying.

Think of all the ads you see on the internet, on TV, or in magazines. They show a cartoon character swallowing a pill. A diagram shows the pill's path down into the stomach. Voila! That is all that it does. People don't stop and realize that all drugs, whether over-the-counter or prescribed, are systemic and have the potential to affect any *and every* part of the body, regardless of the reason you're taking them. Don't believe me? Listen closely to the commercials where the side effects are blurted out quickly with the soft hymn in the background while people run down the beach in the sun. Read all of the horrible side effects written in fine print. Heart problems, breathing problems, DEATH! Open up the leaflet that you get with all your medications. Take out a magnifying glass and read page after page of what can happen.

Unfortunately, most people operate from the "it can't happen to me" part of their brain. But guess what? As time goes on, many people have stories of someone they know who had some reaction to a medication, even if it didn't happen to them personally.

Now, more than ever, people are waking up. People like you are finally asking questions. People like you are finally demanding answers and a different approach. I've been practicing since 2003 and have seen a major shift in how people are thinking for themselves, and I love it. It makes sense that the age of the internet improved our knowledge because people now have as much information at their fingertips as they need and want.

Going back to my story, I took my passion for understanding the human body further and got my bachelor's degree in biology. While in college, I experienced a major pivotal moment in my life that literally changed me forever.

In 2006, I was working for my father in the summertime. Every summer and holiday, I was that hardworking kid who spent more time growing my work ethic than I spent playing. It was August 6. I had taken one day off from working in my dad's factory to go for my annual checkup with my family doctor when I received the fateful call—the call that no one, at any age, especially as young as 19, ever wants to or expects to get. My father had suffered a disastrous stroke, and by the time I made it to the hospital, it was virtually too late.

I remember being by his bedside, feeling hopeless and not being able to process in any way what was taking place. In the blink of an eye, my life was forever altered. My father, my best friend, the man I idolized, was lying there lifeless. He was only fifty-one years old.

How did this all happen? Eventually, after the grieving process—which, as you know, never goes away but does lessen over time—I was able to analyze and evaluate the situation.

I have memories of my father going to the doctor with full-fledged diabetes and blood sugar problems. I remember that his breakfast was an Entenmann's donut with a glass of soda. He never exercised or took care of himself physically. I remember going to the podiatrist with my father and the doctor telling him that his pulses were diminished in his ankles and that he needed to do a 180 for his future.

We all know people like my father. He didn't heed any warning. He didn't want to take charge or take responsibility for his health. He had the thought process that he could continue his poor eating habits because he was taking a medication to cancel out the effects of the new sugar that he was putting into his body. He was operating on the "it can't happen to me" mentality I spoke about earlier.

What did I learn from this? A lot. More than anything, I learned that I didn't want to be like my father. I wanted to be proactive and do everything in my power to take charge of my own health. Even prior to this event, the concept of better health through better chemistry, attained by a lifestyle of pill-popping, never made sense to me. But after all of this, it REALLY made no sense to me. I vowed that my health would be a priority. I would do everything in my power to make the best decisions for what made sense—not what had been brainwashed into me.

The goal is to prevent the health consequences, which my father tucked away in the back of his mind, from even surfacing. To do everything in my power to live a natural, healthy lifestyle, working with my body's ability to heal. To make the correct decisions about what I put into my body if I expect to get amazing things out of it. Exercising regularly to keep my body healthy is essential. Prevention is the key.

It's funny, when you really think about it. The healthcare system we live in isn't really healthcare at all; it's sick-care. When was the last time you went to the doctor to learn how to be *healthy*?

When you go to the doctor, what is the first thing he or she asks you? "Why are you here?" "What hurts?" Or, "What's the problem?" If you said, "Nothing," I think you'd agree that they'd pretty much ask why you're even there. You go to the doctor with a symptom, and they treat that symptom.

Not only was my newfound passion to live a proactive, preventative lifestyle, but I knew it was my calling to help prevent what happened in my life from happening to other people. I wanted to help increase the quality and quantity of peoples' lives, for them and for their families. To help people understand that living your life from the least invasive to the most invasive is ideal. Helping people understand that you should never follow people like sheep in this world, especially when it comes to your health. And don't be afraid to ask questions!

My mission became much bigger than I had ever imagined. It went from understanding how I need to help myself and my family to having an urge to teach and help as many people as possible. This knowledge that I possess needs to be shared. That's why I'm writing this book. I don't expect to change the life of everybody who reads this book, but I do expect to make a difference to most that read it. If I can get you to question things that you've had ingrained in you up until this point when it comes to your health, and open your eyes to making better decisions and actually thinking for yourself, then I am on the way to accomplishing my mission . . . to touch as many lives as I can and make a difference in this world.

Chapter 2: Help Is on the Way

To effectively help you with your neuropathy, you need to understand: There is no cookie cutter treatment. It takes a unique approach by looking at each patient individually. I look at patients like a pizza pie, and your pie is made of three slices.

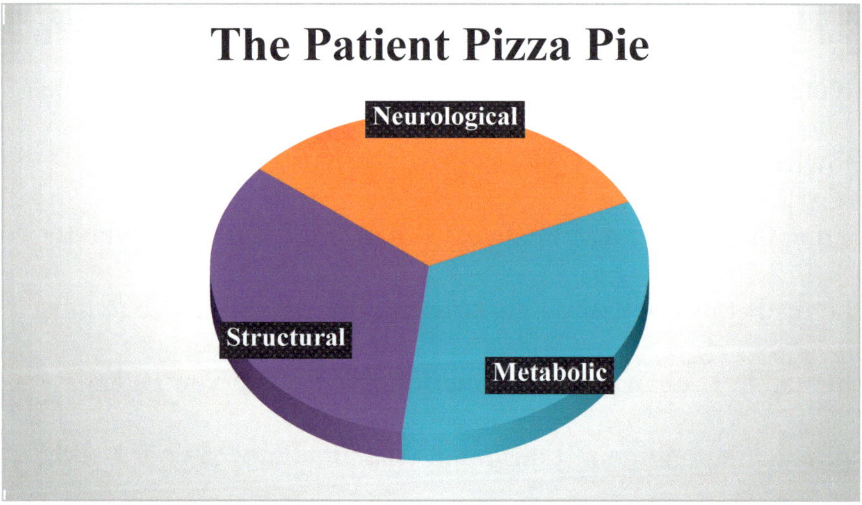

The first slice is your neurology. A thorough evaluation of your nerves and an extensive case history is needed. I care about all my patients, so I spend time with them. I don't have one foot out the door when it comes to patient care, which is, unfortunately, the kind of care most people have become accustomed to. By doing a thorough evaluation, I am able to determine whether I feel your neuropathy symptoms can be helped based upon the level of deterioration that you experience.

The best analogy to give a layperson as to how nerves work is to use the example of an outlet in the wall. If you were to punch a hole in the wall and pull out the wires, you would find that there are multiple wires that do multiple things. When it comes to human nerves, there are different fibers that do different things. Some nerve fibers, when affected, will result in numbness or tingling. Others will result in cramping when the muscle on the other end is involved. And yet another is responsible for temperature issues (for example, not being able to feel the temperature of the water in the shower or feeling hot as cold and cold as hot).

The nerve system in the human body is fascinating and complex, and that's why there are many different presentations of peripheral neuropathy. You could be in a doctor's waiting room with a group of other neuropathy patients, and it would not be at all surprising if none of you were presenting the same symptoms. It's very interesting; neuropathy is like an umbrella diagnosis. What I mean by that is that if you take a common condition in the human body, such as a heart problem, most people suffer from referred pain and chest pain, or pain radiating down the left arm or jaw. If you have a gallbladder problem, you will feel pain referred in the shoulder and in the upper right quadrant of the abdomen. Neuropathy, on the other hand, is its own breed. Since there are so many nerve fibers involved, the function of these nerve fibers determines your symptom presentation. The more symptoms you present with and the greater the intensity of the symptoms . . . the greater the flood.

While on the outside neuropathy patients might all appear the same, in most cases, there are significant differences. It's very common for people to start off with numbness in their toes. Then, over a period of not addressing the root cause of the problems and the nerves, it will start to present with a burn. Then cramps. Then walking on sponges. Then balance issues. Neuropathy is a vicious beast and takes on a life of its own.

After the symptoms intensify, the location spreads. Very often, neuropathy symptoms happen in the tips of the toes, then the toes, then the feet, then up to short socks, then long socks, then leggings, then pants. It's an absolutely horrible condition. Most doctors only attribute it to blood sugar issues, but what if you don't have blood sugar issues? How can that be the only contributing factor resulting in peripheral neuropathy?

The second and third pieces of the pizza pie, after we determine the extent of the nerve damage, are the *whys*. Why is this happening? What led to your problem?

The second piece of the pie is the metabolic piece, which encompasses the physiological causes. I will briefly discuss some of them in this chapter but will go more in-depth in Chapter 5. Blood sugar issues seem to always be the go-to for most doctors. This is the go-to diagnosis because it's the most common, but it's not the only reason! Every cell in your body needs proper glucose *and* proper oxygen to survive, heal, and thrive.

What if you have anemia? What if you have gut (intestinal) issues? 70 to 80 percent of your immune system comes from your digestive tract. FACT. If your gut is not healthy, your immune system will pay the price. When was the last time you healed the tissue of your digestive tract? When was the last time you did a detox for your gut? If we know that it makes up a majority of our immune systems, shouldn't this be of utmost importance?

In addition to blood sugar, anemia, and the gut, what about thyroid issues? Every cell in the human body requires proper levels of thyroid hormone to function well. What about hormonal imbalances and adrenal gland dysfunction? Both can cause chronic inflammation in the tissues of your body—including nerves. And what about food sensitivities? The list goes on. There are many different root causes of peripheral neuropathy proven in peer-reviewed medical journals worldwide AND ones that I see clinically or firsthand in my office every day.

It should be obvious by now that although neuropathy cases may appear different based only on the outside symptoms that you present with, in reality, they are *all* very different cases. In order to see results, you have to evaluate the patient on an individual basis rather than with a cookie-cutter mentality. Everyone is their own unique individual and need to be treated that way. You have to dive into case history, evaluate the nerves appropriately, and find all of the root causes of the patient's condition. Then you have to help those root causes.

In fact, other cases of idiopathic neuropathy can also result from other metabolic dysfunctions besides blood sugar, as stated earlier. Once the neurology is evaluated, the metabolic causes are identified, and any structural issues are found, then you have done a complete evaluation of the individual. It's like a master lock; with the right combination, you can unlock the desired results. *And* just as each case of neuropathy is unique for each individual, the combination is different for every lock.

From a metabolic perspective, one of the most common contributing factors to peripheral neuropathy is diabetes (and other blood sugar problems). The research through the National Institute of Health (NIH) states that 60 to 70 percent of diabetics will develop some form of neuropathy symptoms. However, that same research also indicates that there are many neuropathy cases that are completely unrelated to blood sugar levels. Unfortunately, it seems that in clinical practice, a majority of doctors are overlooking the other root causes, both metabolically and structurally related. They often diagnose these cases as idiopathic, and patients are then left being treated with a medication for their symptoms.

We already know there is no cookie cutter for thoroughly evaluating neuropathy symptoms. A thorough review of the blood work is necessary. In addition, the following form is extremely useful in helping to hone in on what systems are being affected.

That's right—*systems*. Clinically, I have found that most cases of neuropathy where metabolic causes are involved are typically a culmination of more than one health condition, or system, involved. Each category on the form deals with a specific organ system.

Metabolic Assessment Form

Name: ________________________ **Age:** _____ **Sex:** _____ **Date:** ____________

Please list the 5 major health concerns in your order of importance:

1. ____________________
2. ____________________
3. ____________________
4. ____________________
5. ____________________

Please circle the appropriate number "0 - 3" on all questions below. <u>0 as the least/never</u> to <u>3 as the most/always.</u>

Category I

Feeling that bowels do not empty completely	0	1	2	3
Lower abdominal pain relief by passing stool or gas	0	1	2	3
Alternating constipation and diarrhea	0	1	2	3
Diarrhea	0	1	2	3
Constipation	0	1	2	3
Hard, dry, or small stool	0	1	2	3
Coated tongue of "fuzzy" debris on tongue	0	1	2	3
Pass large amount of foul smelling gas	0	1	2	3
More than 3 bowel movements daily	0	1	2	3
Use laxatives frequently	0	1	2	3

Category II

Excessive belching, burping, or bloating	0	1	2	3
Gas immediately following a meal	0	1	2	3
Offensive breath	0	1	2	3
Difficult bowel movements	0	1	2	3
Sense of fullness during and after meals	0	1	2	3
Difficulty digesting fruits and vegetables; undigested foods found in stools	0	1	2	3

Category III

Stomach pain, burning, or aching 1- 4 hours after eating	0	1	2	3
Use antacids	0	1	2	3
Feel hungry an hour or two after eating	0	1	2	3
Heartburn when lying down or bending forward	0	1	2	3
Temporary relief from antacids, food, milk, carbonated beverages	0	1	2	3
Digestive problems subside with rest and relaxation	0	1	2	3
Heartburn due to spicy foods, chocolate, citrus, peppers, alcohol, and caffeine	0	1	2	3

Category IV

Roughage and fiber cause constipation	0	1	2	3
Indigestion and fullness lasts 2-4 hours after eating	0	1	2	3
Pain, tenderness, soreness on left side under rib cage	0	1	2	3
Excessive passage of gas	0	1	2	3
Nausea and/or vomiting	0	1	2	3
Stool undigested, foul smelling, mucous-like, greasy, or poorly formed	0	1	2	3
Frequent urination	0	1	2	3
Increased thirst and appetite	0	1	2	3
Difficulty losing weight	0	1	2	3

Category V

Greasy or high-fat foods cause distress	0	1	2	3
Lower bowel gas and or bloating several hours after eating	0	1	2	3
Bitter metallic taste in mouth, especially in the morning	0	1	2	3
Unexplained itchy skin	0	1	2	3
Yellowish cast to eyes	0	1	2	3
Stool color alternates from clay colored to normal brown	0	1	2	3
Reddened skin, especially palms	0	1	2	3
Dry or flaky skin and/or hair	0	1	2	3
History of gallbladder attacks or stones	0	1	2	3
Have you had your gallbladder removed	Yes	No		

Category VI

Crave sweets during the day	0	1	2	3
Irritable if meals are missed	0	1	2	3
Depend on coffee to keep yourself going or started	0	1	2	3
Get lightheaded if meals are missed	0	1	2	3
Eating relieves fatigue	0	1	2	3
Feel shaky, jittery, or have tremors	0	1	2	3
Agitated, easily upset, nervous	0	1	2	3
Poor memory/forgetful	0	1	2	3
Blurred vision	0	1	2	3

Category VII

Fatigue after meals	0	1	2	3
Crave sweets during the day	0	1	2	3
Eating sweets does not relieve cravings for sugar	0	1	2	3
Must have sweets after meals	0	1	2	3
Waist girth is equal or larger than hip girth	0	1	2	3
Frequent urination	0	1	2	3
Increased thirst and appetite	0	1	2	3
Difficulty losing weight	0	1	2	3

Category VIII

Cannot stay asleep	0	1	2	3
Crave salt	0	1	2	3
Slow starter in the morning	0	1	2	3
Afternoon fatigue	0	1	2	3
Dizziness when standing up quickly	0	1	2	3
Afternoon headaches	0	1	2	3
Headaches with exertion or stress	0	1	2	3
Weak nails	0	1	2	3

Category IX

Cannot fall asleep	0	1	2	3
Perspire easily	0	1	2	3
Under high amounts of stress	0	1	2	3
Weight gain when under stress	0	1	2	3
Wake up tired even after 6 or more hours of sleep	0	1	2	3
Excessive perspiration or perspiration with little or no activity	0	1	2	3

Category X

Tired, sluggish	0	1	2	3
Feel cold – hands, feet, all over	0	1	2	3
Require excessive amounts of sleep to function properly	0	1	2	3
Increase in weight gain even with low-calorie diet	0	1	2	3
Gain weight easily	0	1	2	3
Difficult, infrequent bowel movements	0	1	2	3
Depression, lack of motivation	0	1	2	3
Morning headaches that wear off as the day progresses	0	1	2	3
Outer third of eyebrow thins	0	1	2	3
Thinning of hair on scalp, face, or genitals or excessive falling hair	0	1	2	3
Dryness of skin and/or scalp	0	1	2	3
Mental sluggishness	0	1	2	3

Category XI

Heart palpitations	0	1	2	3
Inward trembling	0	1	2	3
Increased pulse even at rest	0	1	2	3
Nervous and emotional	0	1	2	3
Insomnia	0	1	2	3
Night sweats	0	1	2	3
Difficulty gaining weight	0	1	2	3

Category XII

Diminished sex drive	0	1	2	3
Menstrual disorders or lack of menstruation	0	1	2	3
Increased ability to eat sugars without symptoms	0	1	2	3

Category XIII

Increased sex drive	0	1	2	3
Tolerance to sugars reduced	0	1	2	3
"Splitting" type headaches	0	1	2	3

Category XIV (Males only)

Urination difficulty or dribbling	0	1	2	3
Frequent urination	0	1	2	3
Pain inside of legs or heels	0	1	2	3
Feeling of incomplete bowel evacuation	0	1	2	3
Leg nervousness at night	0	1	2	3

Category XV (Males only)

Decrease in libido	0	1	2	3
Decrease in spontaneous morning erections	0	1	2	3
Decrease in fullness of erections	0	1	2	3
Difficulty in maintaining morning erections	0.	1	2	3
Spells of mental fatigue	0	1	2	3
Inability to concentrate	0	1	2	3
Episodes of depression	0	1	2	3
Muscle soreness	0	1	2	3
Decrease in physical stamina	0	1	2	3
Unexplained weight gain	0	1	2	3
Increase in fat distribution around chest and hips	0	1	2	3
Sweating attacks	0	1	2	3
More emotional than in the past	0	1	2	3

Category XVI (Menstruating Females Only)

Are you perimenopausal	Yes	No		
Alternating menstrual cycle lengths	Yes	No		
Extended menstrual cycle, greater than 32 days	Yes	No		
Shortened menses, less than every 24 days	Yes	No		
Pain and cramping during periods	0	1	2	3
Scanty blood flow	0	1	2	3
Heavy blood flow	0	1	2	3
Breast pain and swelling during menses	0	1	2	3
Pelvic pain during menses	0	1	2	3
Irritable and depressed during menses	0	1	2	3
Acne breakouts	0	1	2	3
Facial hair growth	0	1	2	3
Hair loss/thinning	0	1	2	3

Category XVII (Menopausal Females Only)

How many years have you been menopausal?	________			
Since menopause, do you ever have uterine bleeding?	Yes	No		
Hot flashes	0	1	2	3
Mental fogginess	0	1	2	3
Disinterest in sex	0	1	2	3
Mood swings	0	1	2	3
Depression	0	1	2	3
Painful intercourse	0	1	2	3
Shrinking breasts	0	1	2	3
Facial hair growth	0	1	2	3
Acne	0	1	2	3
Increased vaginal pain, dryness or itching	0	1	2	3

How many alcoholic beverages do you consume per week? ________ How many caffeinated beverages do you consume per day? ________

How many times do you eat out per week? ________ How many times a week do you eat raw nuts or seeds? ________

How many times a week do you eat fish? ________ How many times a week do you workout? ________

List the three worst foods you eat during the average week: ________, ________, ________

List the three healthiest foods you eat during the average week: ________, ________, ________

Do you smoke?______ If yes, how many times a day: ________

Rate your stress levels on a scale of 1-10 during the average week: ________

Please list any medications you currently take and for what conditions:

____

Please list any natural supplements you currently take and for what conditions:

____

Are you left or right handed?	Right	Left
Have you had a head injury?	YES	NO
Do you currently experience or have a past history of vertigo or balance disorders?	YES	NO
Do you have any ringing or pressure in the ears?	YES	NO
Do you experience nausea?	YES	NO
Do you find that your balance is getting worse?	YES	NO
Do you have difficulties walking down stairs?	YES	NO
Do you have difficulty with math problems, or remembering numbers?	YES	NO
Do you find yourself searching for words frequently when you speak?	YES	NO
Have you noticed your ability to concentrate is getting worse?	YES	NO
Do you get lost often or have a hard time with directions?	YES	NO
Do quick flashes of light on TV or loud noises bother you?	YES	NO
Do you feel like you need to wear sunglasses outside?	YES	NO
Has your handwriting changed in recent years?	YES	NO
Do you have a hard time swallowing?	YES	NO
Do you gag easily?	YES	NO
Do you experience blurriness in your vision or double vision? ←(CIRCLE)	YES	NO
Do you have any changes in smell or smell foul things that are not present?	YES	NO
Do you have any difficulty with taste or taste things differently than what you're eating?	YES	NO
Noticed clumsiness in hand coordination? Which hand? Right/Left ←(CIRCLE)	YES	NO

Do you have difficulty with short-term memory?	YES	NO
Have you been told or noticed any memory loss of past events?	YES	NO
Noticed uneven sweating or temperature on one side of your body?	YES	NO
Do you have any tightness, weakness or instability in your back or neck? ←(CIRCLE)	YES	NO
Do you ever have any numbness or tingling in your hands, legs or face? ←(CIRCLE)	YES	NO
Do you have difficulty with falling asleep or staying asleep?	YES	NO
Do you get motion sickness easily (carsick or seasick)?	YES	NO
Do you ever experience flashes of light in your visual field?	YES	NO
Do you ever experience dry eyes or mouth? ←(CIRCLE)	YES	NO
Do you ever experience increase tearing or salivation? ←(CIRCLE)	YES	NO
Do you ever have slurred speech?	YES	NO
Noticed any drooping of your eyelids or facial muscles? ←(CIRCLE)	YES	NO
Do you ever notice increased heart rate (tachycardia) or pulse during the day?	YES	NO
Have you ever experienced or been diagnosed with arrhythmia (fluctuating heart rate)?	YES	NO
Does driving cause you fatigue, headaches, or any other symptoms? ←(CIRCLE)	YES	NO
Does working on a computer cause you fatigue, headaches or other symptoms? ←(CIRCLE)	YES	NO
Have you lost interest in hobbies and functions that you used to enjoy?	YES	NO
Do you have a hard time motivating yourself to engage in activities?	YES	NO
Do you have fluttering of the eye or noticed you are blinking frequently?	YES	NO
Do you have difficulty distinguishing right and left?	YES	NO

It is essential for you to accurately fill out the form in order to determine what further tests are needed. There are many tests available, such as thorough blood panels, stool panels, and saliva panels to help evaluate your health.

In most cases, customized nutritional protocols are necessary to effectively manage neuropathy symptoms. These protocols will be based on the deficiencies uncovered by the thorough analysis. Managing blood sugar levels and insulin resistance is extremely important (see Chapter 6 for samples of dietary protocols often used with neuropathy patients). Specific nutritional products are typically recommended in order to help the body recover. All of these are based on your individual needs.

The third piece of the pizza pie is structure. The nerves that go down your legs to your feet come from your lower back and cross through a knee and ankle joint to get to your feet. If you develop a spinal condition, such as disc issues or stenosis, these conditions can have extreme relevance to your peripheral neuropathy. These cases are often described as "idiopathic" in the medical world, meaning that the symptoms arose spontaneously. If you hear this word, it simply means that your doctors are baffled as to why you have the symptoms that you do, despite the fact that you DON'T have blood sugar issues.

There are also many cases of neuropathy in the legs and feet post-surgical intervention. I have seen cases that began after knee surgery and/or replacement, hip surgery, ankle surgery, and other variations of leg surgery. In the next chapter, we'll discuss neuropathy in more detail and its effects on overall health.

Chapter 3: How Much Worse Can I Get?

At this point, you may be wondering, what are the common consequences when a neuropathy condition is left untreated over time?

Balance is absolutely the most important out of all of the associated concerns. Every second of every day in the United States, an older adult falls, making falls the number one cause of injuries and deaths from injury among older Americans. In 2014 alone, older Americans experienced 29 million falls, causing seven million injuries and costing an estimated $31 billion in annual Medicare costs, according to a new Morbidity and Mortality Weekly Report (MMWR) published by the Centers for Disease Control and Prevention.

"Older adult falls are increasing and, sadly, often herald the end of independence," said CDC Director Tom Frieden, M.D., M.P.H. "Healthcare providers can make fall prevention a routine part of care in their practice, and older adults can take steps to protect themselves."

With more than 10,000 older Americans turning 65 each day, the number of fall-related injuries and deaths is expected to surge, resulting in cost increases unless preventive measures are taken.

Can you imagine your neuropathy affecting you to the point that you need an assisted walking device such as a cane or walker? Picture this: You're walking through the grocery store and need to sit down while your loved one continues to shop because you can't keep up. You used to be the one who set the pace, and now you're the one that slows the pace.

What happens if your lifestyle completely changes, and you lose the ability to do the things you enjoy? Let's say you like to golf on the weekends, but you're developing some numbness or tingling in your feet. Most people in this situation have to walk and stand wider in stature to provide more stability while on their feet. When you play golf, that numbness or tingling in your feet will affect your stance, as you will not feel comfortable having your feet in a narrow position beneath your shoulders. This can certainly affect your balance, how you twist your body when you swing, and how you drive the ball. Many golfers report having difficulty walking on unsteady surfaces such as the green, and even state how insecure they feel getting up and down out of the cart. This can be devastating to an avid golfer who has spent years playing with friends. Can you imagine having to hang up your clubs, not being able to play golf with those friends ever again? The sooner you seek help for your neuropathy and the more proactive you are, the better chance you have to continue doing the activities that you enjoy.

Shifting from the green to the court, tennis is another sport that many people enjoy—and hope to enjoy for life. But tennis players also have concerns when it comes to their neuropathy. They typically report difficulty with the stop and go of the game. When your feet lose perception and you are unable to detect the ground well underneath your feet, you can feel extremely unsteady and susceptible to a fall. It's common that the fear of falling takes over and leads to a decline in the speed of your game to the point that you find it difficult to consider yourself a competitor anymore. Eventually, it can lead to giving up on the game altogether, as it is no longer found to be enjoyable and poses too great a risk.

Chronic neuropathy patients reach the point when they are incapable of taking care of themselves. Eventually, even the task of driving becomes extremely difficult because they are unable to effectively detect the gas pedal or the brake. I've had patients report that they had to stop driving because they were not able to confidently stop their car. They were relying on the pressure of the brake pedal pushing back at them and were purposefully stopping about 200 feet behind the car in front of them, just to comfortably stop at a light.

The reaction time of a neuropathy patient becomes a significant problem when driving a vehicle, as many patients report that it becomes difficult for the feet to be responsive to what their brain is telling them. The more the nerves are affected, the more severe this issue becomes. Cases of neuropathy that afflict the upper extremities and hands can also affect driving. The tactile sense of gripping and feeling the steering wheel becomes diminished.

All of the above aspects of affected driving pose risks not only to the person driving but to other people on the road. Patients who proactively identify this difficulty and come to terms with the fact that they shouldn't be driving should be commended. It takes a certain level of acknowledgment for someone, who has been driving for potentially decades and decades, to come to the understanding that it is no longer safe to do so. At this point, the responsibility gets shifted to the spouse.

Dependence on others is a major side effect of neuropathy. Patients get to the point that their mobility is so affected that they can't do the things that they love to do, and they become dependent upon others. Can you imagine how much your life changes when your neuropathy gets so severe that your ability to complete your daily tasks is dependent on someone else? This is extremely difficult for most patients to process. From a psychological standpoint, it is common for neuropathy patients to exhibit some form of depression. No one likes to feel dependent.

So, what is the key to avoiding this? Do everything in your power to avoid getting to this point.

I see patients who need help walking around their own home they've lived in for thirty years. They need help going to the bathroom, bathing, and getting dressed, especially when their balance is affected. I've seen cases where neuropathy affects the hands in such a way that the person loses the ability to hold a toothbrush, use a razor, open a jar of peanut butter, or even distinguish the difference between a dime or a nickel in their wallet.

I find it extremely upsetting when someone has spent their entire life working hard to get to the point that they are able to retire, only to find themselves unable to do the things that they retired to be able to do in the first place. Losing your enjoyment after a life of hard work is no way to spend your golden years.

Helping patients achieve the results that they're looking for with their neuropathy symptoms is extremely satisfying. Giving someone the capability to resume the activities that they are passionate about is as gratifying as it gets.

What Else Can Peripheral Neuropathy Lead To?

From a clinical standpoint, peripheral neuropathy can potentially lead to and/or contribute to a variety of other health conditions. Most commonly, neuropathy symptoms affect the joints. They can intensify existing chronic knee conditions, as well as contribute to new knee conditions.

How is that so? Let me connect the dots of what I see clinically with a vivid image from my childhood.

I used to ride to work with my father in Maspeth, Queens. I remember my father driving down Maspeth Avenue going literally at five miles per hour because the potholes were the size of children. I would hear the car squeak and make noises in places that I didn't even know existed. What those roads did to the shocks of our car that we drove on a daily basis was devastating. Think about it. Let's suppose the shocks on our car were destroyed, and we went to the mechanic for new shocks. What would happen if we continued driving down that same bumpy road? Exactly. The new shocks would deteriorate just as quickly.

This analogy is extremely relevant to what can happen to the knees of a neuropathy patient. If your lower legs and feet are the sensors to the ground underneath you, but you are unable to detect the ground due to peripheral nerves that are losing or altering their perception, your knees receive the brunt of the force.

When you lose perception in your lower legs and feet, however, your brain has options. First, you can suffer a fall from the loss or altered perception. The brain wants to avoid this at any cost. Remember, falling is now the number one cause of death in the older population. Therefore, the brain can choose to compensate in order to maintain stability. These compensations often affect the knee joints.

There are scenarios where patients overplant their feet with every step that they take in a day. Think about the hundreds, if not thousands, of steps that the average person takes in one day. A neuropathy patient may overplant their feet with every step they take to exaggerate the force and perception of the ground underneath them. With more impact, the brain can better perceive the ground. However, this is done at the cost of the shock-absorbing knee joints.

Just as the knee joints can be impacted by neuropathy in the feet, knee replacement surgery can also lead to nerve issues. When a knee replacement surgery is performed, the lower leg is literally detached and reattached with a replacement joint and hardware. It is common to see patients with nerves that are affected just from this surgery alone. Visit YouTube to watch a video of a knee surgery with your own two eyes.

The same abnormal pressure that can be applied to the knees due to loss or altered perception can also be related to ankle injuries. Both the knees and the ankles are weight-bearing joints and are directly dependent upon the foundation below them and the actions of the feet.

Plantar fasciitis is also seen clinically with neuropathy patients in my office. The plantar fascia is the connective tissue from the ball of the foot to the heel, on the bottom of your foot. This foot pain can become so debilitating that it, in and of itself, can disable a patient. Patients who suffer from plantar fasciitis find it very difficult to stand or walk for long periods of time, and they can even have difficulty wearing shoes. The reason that this condition is correlated to neuropathy conditions is no different than what was stated above regarding knees and ankles. As a neuropathy patient with lost or diminished perception overplants their feet to better help them detect the ground underneath them, the tissues on the bottom of the feet absorb a tremendous amount of pressure. Over time, this can lead to chronically inflamed tissue on the bottom of the foot, which is known as plantar fasciitis.

Lower back pain can often result from peripheral neuropathy in the feet, just as it can contribute to neuropathy in the feet. The nerves that go down the legs to the feet come from the lower back. If disc issues or stenosis are present and the nerves are being affected at the spinal level, (the fuse box of your body), peripheral neuropathy can certainly result. This is typically a factor involved in the cases where patients are diagnosed with idiopathic neuropathy, as stated earlier. However, the mechanics of the lower back can also be directly and negatively influenced by the loss of perception and altered gait patterns that accompany a neuropathy condition.

If a neuropathy patient has any change in their mobility and stature, such as walking while leaning more to one side or more forward than they should, this can eventually lead to abnormal weight distribution in the hips, lower back, and pelvis. When the joints involved in these areas are asymmetrically loaded over time, it can cause a mechanical breakdown, and your biomechanics pay the price. Chronic pain and even further change in stature and gait pattern can ensue.

The way the feet can affect the ankle—which can affect a knee, which can affect a hip, which can affect a lower back—is traditionally referred to as a safety pin cycle. Just as the song goes, "The hip bone's connected to the leg bone." (Did you just sing that too?) Every part of what we call the lower extremity kinetic chain is dependent upon one another.

By the way, what has always frustrated me personally—and now professionally, on behalf of patients—is that you can go to your doctor with a complaint about a body part within your kinetic chain yet literally never have your kinetic chain evaluated.

Let's say you go to the traditional doctor with a knee complaint, for example. You're unlikely to receive the thorough analysis that you deserve, because the doctor will only be focused on your knee symptoms. Unless you have an ache or pain in another specific area, your doctor will *only* look at the knee, not the entire biomechanical system.

Why are patients with knee problems not having their entire extremities (kinetic chains) evaluated? The knee has an influence on the hips and lower back above, as well as the ankles and feet below. It seems as though these doctors literally wait for someone to deteriorate enough to have a symptom manifest before it is even investigated. I believe in being more proactive than that and take a complete preventative approach by evaluating the chief complaint as well as what else could be involved and influenced. That's what I call thorough, personalized care that every human being deserves. In Chapter 7, I'll share how *you* can get exactly that. But first, let's talk about functional medicine—WHY this is happening to you and HOW you got here.

Chapter 4: Get the Results

What if I told you that it was possible to get the results that you are looking for? Maybe you're one of the innumerable patients who have been told that there's nothing you can do. You just have to live with your symptoms. It simply comes with age, and once nerves die, you can't help them anymore.

But what if your doctors are wrong?

Your doctors are giving their opinion based upon their thought processes and the tools that are available in their toolbox. If all you have is a hammer, every problem looks like a nail. Any project that requires a saw, screwdriver, or pair of pliers will, of course, never work.

These doctors do a great job with acute emergency care. The medications that they use for peripheral neuropathy are their "hammers." But did you know that these medications were originally used as anti-seizure medications, which are useful for *slowing down the brain*? The reason these drugs are effective for neuropathy patients is because they affect how the brain perceives the symptoms of peripheral nerve damage. Nothing at all is done for *treating* the deteriorating nerve itself. Therefore, if all the doctor does is give you an anti-seizure medication, then it is possibly accurate that you cannot be helped. There aren't any surgeries that would help deteriorating peripheral nerves, either.

But what if you were able to proactively help the nerves? If you shifted gears from a symptom-oriented mindset to a mindset of looking for a root cause to identify the problem, you would see that there are better and far more effective options.

This is why it is important to focus on the metabolic component, as discussed earlier. A thorough review of your labs is essential. As stated earlier, blood sugar is the most common contributor to neuropathy, but is by far not the only one. A complete thyroid panel (beyond TSH and T4), anemia, in-depth immune system function, digestive health, hormones, and adrenal gland function are all necessary to accurately determine the health of any individual. It's also important to look at the values on bloodwork from a functional medicine standpoint.

What is functional medicine? The Institute for Functional Medicine defines it as follows.

"Functional Medicine addresses the underlying causes of disease, using a systems-oriented approach and engaging both patient and practitioner in a therapeutic partnership. It is an evolution in the practice of medicine that better addresses the healthcare needs of the twenty-first century. By shifting the traditional disease-centered focus of medical practice to a more patient-centered approach, Functional Medicine addresses the whole person, not just an isolated set of symptoms. Functional Medicine practitioners spend time with their patients, listening to their histories and looking at the interactions among genetic, environmental, and lifestyle factors that can influence long-term health and complex, chronic disease. In this way, Functional Medicine supports the unique expression of health and vitality for each individual."

There are six core principles in functional medicine.

1. An understanding of the biochemical individuality of each human being, based on the concepts of genetic and environmental uniqueness
2. Awareness of the evidence that supports a patient-centered rather than a disease-centered approach to treatment

3. Search for a dynamic balance among the internal and external body, mind, and spirit
4. Interconnections of internal physiological factors
5. Identification of health as a positive vitality, not merely the absence of disease, and emphasizing those factors that encourage the enhancement of a vigorous physiology
6. Promotion of organ reserve as the means to enhance the health span, not just the lifespan, of each patient.

The future of healthcare will be treating in every patient as an individual, no longer by lumping the patient into the group of symptoms that make up a named disease process. The conventional habit of generalized symptom care will slowly shift over to accurate and specific care for each patient.

Not only does this new system make sense, but the public is aware—now more than ever—and is demanding this type of treatment. Look at the trend of frustrated doctors and patients who are opting for concierge offices. If you've never heard of this type of office, it's when doctors choose to opt out of insurance-based practices in order to provide the quality of care that they prefer. They charge the patient a flat fee to reserve them as a doctor for the year so that the patient can get more personalized care.

This trend emerged because doctors were getting so overwhelmed, as they needed to see almost twice as many patients to make up for the loss of insurance reimbursements. Doctors running concierge offices are no longer forced to follow the dictated orders of insurance companies and are now able to focus on what a patient actually needs, not what the usual and customary tests are for certain symptoms. For example, in the past, if a patient came in with Problem A, doctors were *only* able to run tests that were known to possibly correlate with Problem A, according to the regulating insurance companies. On the contrary, now doctors can get back to focusing on doing a comprehensive workup and helping their patients get better.

Functional medicine fits into this paradigm very well. Doctors are being forced to go back to the anatomy and physiology that they learned about and understand the body as a whole again, as was once practiced in the past—understanding that Problem A and Problem B on the first page of the blood work are actually the results of Process C and Process D on the second page.

Rather than popping a pill for every symptom, functional medicine gets back to investigating and understanding the WHY. Why is this happening? Where is this coming from? Functional medicine operates with the thought process that every single person is their own intricate puzzle. It's the doctor's job to piece together the puzzle. Think about it. For just about every condition that you know of in the human body, there can be a multitude of reasons why something is taking place. And for every person with the same diagnosis, there can actually be complete different WHYs. Now, let's discuss the HOWs.

Chapter 5: How Did You Get Here? Is It Still Going On?

Identifying all the root causes of your health issues, from a physiological perspective, is imperative. You need to get down to the WHY to help to change it for the better. Now, let's talk about a couple of examples of metabolic roots of neuropathy and get specific on HOW they contribute to the problem. . . .

First, there are blood sugar problems, also known as dysglycemia.

High blood sugar interferes with the ability of the nerves to transmit signals. It also weakens the walls of the small blood vessels (capillaries) that supply the nerves with oxygen and nutrients. On the other hand, something that is almost *never* spoken about is low blood sugar. Too little oxygen and nutrients being supplied to the nerves is also a problem.

In the world of functional medicine, the appropriate range of healthy blood sugar is 85–99. Above that is too high, and below that is too low. A person is classified as having diabetes when their blood sugar is higher than 130. Between 100 and 129, you are considered insulin-resistant. It is much easier to address dysglycemia *before* it becomes a diagnosed diabetic condition.

More important than blood glucose is the hemoglobin A1C value. A1C is frequently used to help newly diagnosed diabetics determine how elevated their uncontrolled blood glucose levels have been over the last two to three months. A nondiabetic person will have an A1C result of less than 5.7 percent (39 mmol/mol). Therefore, that is the range to strive for.

How Does Anemia Contribute to Neuropathy?

If a patient has low iron levels, that also means that the production of hemoglobin decreases. Without hemoglobin, red blood cells cannot function, and oxygen levels will drop in the body.

Every cell in the human body needs proper glucose AND proper oxygen levels to function properly, including nerve cells. Iron deficiency anemia is an example of a type of anemia that can result in peripheral neuropathy. A diet that lacks iron, folic acid (folate), or vitamin B12 can prevent your body from making enough red blood cells and supplying proper oxygen to the nerve cells. Further, a deficiency of iron can affect nerve conduction, and a lack of vitamin B12 can damage the myelin sheath that surrounds and protect nerves.

Neuropathy Can Be Caused by Common Medications You May Be Taking

Examples of these medications are:

Heart or blood pressure drugs

- Hydralazine
- Amiodarone
- Perhexiline

Anticonvulsants (phenytoin)

Drugs used to fight cancer

- Docetaxel
- Cisplatin
- Paclitaxel
- Vincristine
- Suramin

Drugs used to fight infections

- Metronidazole (Flagyl)
- Chloroquine
- Nitrofurantoin
- Isoniazid (INH), used against tuberculosis
- Thalidomide (used to fight leprosy)

Drugs used to treat autoimmune disease

- Infliximab
- Etanercept
- Leflunomide

Drugs used to treat skin conditions (Dapsone)

Anti-alcohol drugs (Disulfiram)

Drugs to fight HIV

- Didanosine (Videx)
- Stavudine (Zerit)
- Zalcitabine (Hivid)

Drugs used to treat Cancer

Chemotherapy and radiation are also causes of neuropathy. These are the usual and customary treatment options for saving someone's life from cancer, but unfortunately, some level of neuropathy results since all aspects of the human body are affected.

Colchicine

Arsenic

Hopefully, a light bulb is coming on above your head, and you're starting to understand how complicated neuropathy can be and why every case is unique in its own way, even if, on the outside, they appear identical.

Chronic Inflammation Has Been Linked to Nerve Damage

Neuritis is the medical term for nerve inflammation. When inflammation is affecting a group of nerves, the appropriate term is *polyneuritis*. Nerve inflammation can be caused by numerous health conditions such as:

- Diabetes mellitus
- Autoimmune diseases, ex: lupus, colitis, Crohn's disease, celiac disease, Hashimoto's encephalopathy, multiple sclerosis
- Infections, e.g., herpes zoster, chickenpox, meningitis, viral encephalitis, bacterial pneumonia, and upper respiratory tract infections to name a few
- Metabolic issues
- Malnutrition—vitamin B-12 deficiency
- Neurotoxins, insecticides, mercury, lead, arsenic, alcohol
- Chronic acidosis
- Bell's palsy
- Guillain-Barre syndrome
- Bone fracture, dislocation, herniated disc
- Physical trauma, penetrating injury, bad bruise, heavy pressure on a nerve

Hormonal Imbalances Have Been Shown to Contribute to Neuropathy Conditions

This can occur, whether it's an increase in cortisol production from the adrenal glands, a decrease in thyroid hormones, or a decrease in estrogen levels in postmenopausal women. The hormones are part of our endocrine system, and when this system is involved, it can greatly alter metabolic processes throughout the body.

Changes in cortisol production can have disastrous effects on the human body. This hormone is produced in the adrenal glands, is known as the "stress hormone" and is responsible for the "fight or flight" response in your body—when you're trying to get out of danger, for example. The more emotional, physical, or chemical stress that someone is under, the more dysregulated their cortisol will become.

Do you know anyone under a lot of stress? Of course you do! Unfortunately, stress is a large part of everyone's lives and can lead to significant problems. Cortisol problems have been directly correlated with the following problems in the body:

- Blood sugar imbalances and obesity
- Weight gain and obesity—are you unable to shake the weight no matter how much you exercise or eat appropriately?
- Gastrointestinal problems
- Cardiovascular disease
- Fertility problems
- Immune system suppression
- Chronic fatigue syndrome
- Thyroid issues
- Insomnia

- Depression

The most effective way to evaluate cortisol levels is through an ASI (adrenal stress index). In the functional medicine world, this is done using a saliva panel. If a conventional medical practitioner were to even tests the adrenal glands, they would use the typical method of blood work, but these saliva panel kits can be provided by a health professional and will effectively evaluate adrenal function. The ASI will be able to show what stage of adrenal fatigue you are in, and the skilled practitioner will help you based upon your lab data. One of the main reasons saliva is used instead of blood is because it is pertinent to assess how the adrenal glands are working over a period of time throughout the day. The saliva panel takes into account four readings for the day, whereas blood work only shows data at one moment in time.

Food Sensitivities Can Result in Neuropathy Conditions

Food sensitivities can trigger an immune response in the body as well as a heightened state of inflammation. Peer-reviewed medical journals worldwide have linked autoimmune conditions to gluten, soy, dairy, and egg exposure when an individual possesses an allergy to these foods.

When you ingest foods you are allergic to, it triggers an immune response in your body beginning in the digestive tract. Continued exposure to these allergens can result in a condition known as "leaky gut syndrome." In cases where sensitivities or leaky gut exist, it is absolutely essential to detoxify and heal the tissue in the digestive tract. There are specific protocols that I use with patients to heal their digestive tract and help get them the results that they're looking for.

Chapter 6: Make the Change!

At this point, you may be wondering, how can you make a change in metabolic function if physiological problems are leading to the neuropathy? It all starts with nutrition and lifestyle. The classic saying is, "Garbage in equals garbage out." What you put in your body is what you receive.

One of the most effective dietary regimens to help patients with neuropathy is one focusing on increasing immune system function and decreasing inflammation. It is very important to have a dietary regimen that contains a healthy source of quality protein, healthy fats, vegetables, and fruits. Avoiding carbohydrates, sugars, and complex carbohydrates is crucial. It's very important to start off with a preliminary assessment to determine exactly what you are eating. I always advise patients to start the dietary modification process by filling out the following form:

Name: ______________________________ **Date:** __________

Daily Food Log

Day 1

Time: ____________

Breakfast: ______________________________

____

Time: ____________

Snack: ______________________________

____

Time: ____________

Lunch: ______________________________

____

Time: ____________

Snack: ______________________________

____

Time: ____________

Dinner: ______________________________

____

Name: ______________________________ **Date:** ____________

Daily Food Log

Day 2

Time: ____________

Breakfast: ____

____

Time: ____________

Snack: ____

____

Time: ____________

Lunch: ____

____

Time: ____________

Snack: ____

____

Time: ____________

Dinner: ____

____

Name: ______________________________ **Date:** ____________

Daily Food Log

Day 3

Time: ____________

Breakfast: ______________________________

____

____

Time: ____________

Snack: ______________________________

____

Time: ____________

Lunch: ______________________________

____

Time: ____________

Snack: ______________________________

____

Time: ____________

Dinner: ______________________________

____

When I advise patients on nutrition, it is vital to discuss one very important concept. In helping patients with extremely chronic conditions, it's imperative to understand that there are four main foods that may need to be avoided. These four main foods can potentially contribute to inflammatory and/or destructive processes in the body when you are sensitive or allergic to them.

Those four foods are:

- Gluten
- Soy
- Dairy
- Eggs

The only way to know if you are sensitive or allergic to these foods is to truly test for them. There are numerous ways of doing this through highly reputable labs that look at blood and stool samples. I always encourage patients to perform this testing so that they know for the rest of their life what belongs—or doesn't belong—in their bodies.

Don't you think you need to know this stuff? Not only is it essential to your health, but it's also important because certain food sensitivities are genetic and can affect your loved ones. Getting the results that you are looking for entails claiming responsibility for your own health and being proactive with testing for foods that may cause you harm. You only get this one life, so you must take care of yourself. No one else will ever value your health and well-being the way you should!

If you have a sensitivity to one or more of the foods mentioned above, things may seem complicated. From working with patients on a regular basis, I have noticed that people tend to get confused and discouraged, so instead, let's talk about what you *can* eat—not what you *can't*—from here on.

What Can I Eat?

A lot of the stress of dietary change comes from telling a person what they can't do, especially when it's something that they've done a certain way for many years. I'm going to prove to you that what we're discussing IS possible, and it's actually easier than you think. Let's get started by talking about what is fair game. I think you'll be pleasantly surprised once I explain it to you.

Every meal—breakfast, lunch, and dinner—should consist of a protein. What constitutes a healthy protein? Fish (limited to several times throughout the week), turkey, chicken, veal, pork, and even red meat are all viable options. Yes, you heard me—even red meat. As long as you eat red meat in moderation, it's fair game. Lean meats are important because they are filled with important nutrients like B vitamins (thiamin, B6, niacin, riboflavin), which are important for our nervous system health and metabolism, and they assist in red blood cell formation. Lean meats also contain iron, which helps maintain energy and carry oxygen through the bloodstream; magnesium, which is vital for building bones; and zinc, which is essential for our immune system.

Protein

One question that may be coming to your mind right now is, if I told you to avoid eggs, and if you choose to test for them, what can you eat for breakfast? It's funny. The ingrained, Americanized diet that we've been brainwashed into thinking is appropriate—from watching TV as youngsters and seeing ads in magazines—is the typical box of cereal, a pitcher of milk, orange juice, and a pair of over-easy eggs. Therefore, patients often ask me what they can eat for breakfast if they can't have eggs.

Don't be fooled by the old, American breakfast mindset. Other cultures have no problem eating leftovers from the night before, such as some of their rotisserie chicken, or even having red meat for breakfast. This concept seems to be difficult for most people to understand because it's out of their comfort zones of what they feel is usual and customary. If you don't want to adopt the leftovers mentality of consuming other types of protein for breakfast, certainly a viable option is a protein shake.

The next question usually is, "What type of protein shake should I use?" Have you ever heard of whey protein? No way, no whey. It is common for people to have an allergy to whey without even knowing. I recommend beef protein, since we are carnivores, as proven by our digestive tracts and the structure of our teeth. I know some vegans may be reading this book, so other options are pea protein or hemp protein if you would prefer to avoid the beef protein route. A great way to prepare a protein shake is to use a base of almond milk (since I'm recommending that you avoid dairy, as previously discussed). Add berries such as blueberries, blackberries, raspberries, or strawberries and also some green vegetables or a green powdered nutritional supplement. This is a great, nutritious breakfast that will start the day off on the right path.

Vegetables

Vegetables are extremely important and are the most neglected foods of those suggested. Let's face it, people never really have a problem consuming fruit. After all, fruits are delicious because of all of the natural sugar that they have. However, it is recommended that your vegetable intake should be larger than your fruit intake. What constitutes a healthy vegetable? I recommend sticking to green, leafy vegetables such as spinach, kale, broccoli, asparagus, bok choy, cucumbers, celery, avocado, and brussels sprouts to name a few. Leafy green vegetables are full of vitamins, minerals, and disease-fighting phytochemicals, which lower your risk of type 2 diabetes and cardiovascular disease. Vegetables that you want to avoid are the nightshade vegetables. This term describes vegetables that are grown in the shade or that flower at night. Tomatoes, eggplants, potatoes, and peppers are examples. These should be avoided because in some people, they can trigger an immune reaction similar to a gluten or dairy allergy, which can contribute to autoimmune conditions, leaky gut, or other gut-related illnesses.

Fruits

What constitutes a healthy fruit? I always recommend sticking with the berries such as blackberries, raspberries, blueberries, and strawberries. Specifically, raspberries contain ellagic acid, a compound that contains anti-cancer properties, and blueberries contain powerful antioxidants called anthocyanins, that may help keep memory sharp as you age. All berries are great sources of polyphenols, which may increase levels of nitric oxide, a molecule that can help cardiovascular health by relaxing blood vessels, lowering blood pressure and improving heart health. Polyphenols also contain anthocyanins and ellagic acid, which provides anti-cancer properties and antioxidants for memory. Polyphenols have also been shown in studies to preserve bone density loss after menopause. The outstanding research for the many health benefits of berries continues to grow and prove their power.

If you're a diabetic, the absolute worst fruit that you can eat for blood sugar purposes is a banana. They are the highest of all fruits on the glycemic index, the method for ranking the effects of carbohydrates on blood sugar levels. Apples, berries, grapefruit, prunes, pears, plums, and citrus fruits are lower on the glycemic index. Also high on the glycemic index are melons, raisins, and mangoes. The higher the glycemic value, the more it can affect blood sugar levels. Therefore, the high glycemic fruits listed should be avoided by diabetics and insulin-resistant patients, since they will send your blood sugar on an unhealthy roller coaster ride.

Vegetables and fruits are both extremely important for the antioxidant powers that they provide by building up your immune system. Antioxidants help to protect your body's cells from the potential harm posed by free radicals, which are hazardous molecules produced as byproducts when your body breaks down food or is exposed to tobacco smoke or radiation. Heart disease, cancer, and other diseases have been linked to free radical production in the body.

When to Eat

One of the most important things that people tend to overlook—and something that's just as important as eating the correct foods—is eating them at correct times of the day. For example, if you eat breakfast at 8:00 a.m., lunch at 12:00 p.m., and dinner at 6:30 p.m., snacks between meals should absolutely be incorporated around 10:00 a.m. and 3:00 p.m.

One main reason for consistency of meals is for appropriate blood sugar regulation. When you don't eat at appropriate times and have too much time between meals, your body will produce excess cortisol to regulate your blood sugar. Cortisol is a huge PRO-inflammatory hormone and can cause issues with all tissues in the body, including nerves.

Are you one of those people who struggle with losing weight despite eating healthy, and no matter how much you exercise? The same cortisol problem that I refer to above can also be the reason why you can't shake the weight. Not only is cortisol a major pro-inflammatory, it is also a major fat-producing hormone. Cortisol is absolutely necessary in the human body in sufficient quantities, but not too high or too low. In reality, if you really think about it, isn't that the case with *everything* in the body? Just like Goldilocks—not too high, not too low, but just right.

What we have focused on above is the metabolic and nutritional component of optimizing how your body heals and how to help improve most health conditions. If you remember the pizza pie analogy that we spoke about at the beginning of the book, you'll recall that you also need to focus on the neurological and structural components of your condition.

There are certain treatment methods that I have used in practice for years that help to improve nerve function. If structure is involved, such as spinal disc issues, spinal stenosis, or previous knee surgeries, those scenarios need to be addressed as well. There are high-octane devices and treatments in my office that I use on an individualized, case-by-case basis.

The purpose of this book was to open your eyes to how complicated peripheral neuropathy can be and to show you how you can help yourself at home. Although many people can suffer from the same symptomatic presentation, I'm sure it's very clear to you now that the cases can be completely different based upon the root causes.

Now, your eyes are opened to the fact that in order to optimize your results, *you* are responsible for applying what I have introduced to you. Up until this point, it's quite possible that the only course of action you have taken has been symptomatic care through medication and a protocol of merely monitoring your condition. But now, you know better. I know you deserve the best when it comes to your health, and you need to know all of the options that are available to you.

I have seen the world change since I entered practice in 2003. I used to do workshops to educate patients about nutrition and to share ways that they could help themselves at home. In some instances, it was like pulling teeth, and in many instances, it was a battle. Often, patients wanted to run the information by their family or friends first. They wanted to check with their doctors—who never understood the concepts discussed here to begin with—or even the eighteen-year-old working at the nutrition store, pushing the monthly incentive product.

Once the internet started to explode and you were able to get a world of information at your fingertips, things began to change. Now, people are demanding answers. Patients are questioning their doctors more frequently, since they now have exposure to more knowledge than they have ever had, as they should. The internet has provided a platform where no one needs to be left in the dark anymore, and knowledge can spread like wildfire.

Whether it's a website focusing on the human body, a patient researching the drugs that they've been prescribed, or even a blog from someone across the globe that is introducing a new concept that you've never heard of, there is constantly a surplus of information. Of course, take what you learn and discuss it with the arsenal of doctors who you trust with your health decisions. But understand that now more than ever, YOU have a say, and you should never feel lost.

Chapter 7: Take Back Control

So, what have we learned?

Hopefully, my personal story has given you some new insights on peripheral neuropathy. Not only is this disease much more common than most people realize, but the presentation of symptoms can differ vastly from person to person. My objective with this book was to pass on the knowledge I've gained from my many years of clinical practice. I truly hope that your eyes have been opened and that you will help spread the word to others.

The growing accessibility of information, thanks to the internet, has allowed patients and family members to take their health into their own hands like never before, but there's still a glaring lack of awareness when it comes to this widespread and debilitating health concern. When you take into account peripheral neuropathy symptoms such chronic pain, numbness, falls among the elderly, and the eventual inability of patients to take care of themselves, it's clear that this is a serious issue in need of more effective intervention and treatment.

As you've learned from this book, traditional doctors—who are primarily focused on disease care and symptom-relief—may misattribute neuropathy symptoms to only being from diabetes, insulin resistance, or other blood sugar issues. Instead of associating Problem A and Problem B as the results of Process C, doctors just prescribe whatever medications are recommended for treating Problems A and B, effectively ignoring the process that caused them in the first place. Worse still, they may prescribe neuropathy patients with anti-seizure medicines that slow down the brain. This may certainly ease symptoms, but it will do nothing to fix the actual underlying problem.

The question is, now that you know the truth, where do you go from here? What do you do now?

By applying the "pizza pie" approach and its three categories (neurological, metabolic, and structural), you can manage your peripheral neuropathy symptoms, instead of simply trying to mask the symptoms. We've learned that detoxing the body is not just beneficial but arguably essential to overall health. We have learned that many common medications can cause neuropathy symptoms.

We've also learned about the danger of food sensitivities, the importance of diet, and how specific changes to your food intake can have a major impact on your overall health, including your nervous system. You now know what to eat, when to eat it, and why, and I've given you the resources to log your food intake and monitor the results. Plus, with the Metabolic Assessment Form I've included, you can track and self-evaluate your symptoms, which is the first step toward determining if in-depth testing is needed.

But perhaps most importantly, we've learned that health is not simply the absence of disease. Your health is not a laundry list of symptoms. We must return to a place of understanding the human body as a whole. As such, your first step toward vitality is to shift from a traditional disease-centered view of healthcare to a functional medicine approach—to see every person as an individual composed of vital, interconnected processes, all held in a dynamic balance that creates a unique human being, different from anyone else on Earth.

Now comes the hard part: applying all this new knowledge and *doing* something about it!

What I've learned in life is that it's very easy to gather information but much harder to take the next step to initiate and implement the change. *Step up!* Take charge of your health! No one will EVER value your health as much as you do.

Knowledge without action is absolutely useless. The definition of insanity is doing the same thing over and over again, expecting a different result. If treating symptoms is your only course of action for any health condition that you suffer from, then you are continuing to neglect the root cause. Healthcare should be more than just generalized symptom care. With the knowledge you've gained from this book and the resources I've supplied, you can reject the disease-centered paradigm of healthcare.

It's time—probably the first time in your life—to take charge of your own health. Do what makes sense to you, and always go with your gut. However, I implore you to educate yourself and take the initiative to not just learn "both sides of the fence" but the entire property. Your knowledge should cover as much real estate as possible! Make sure that you work with healthcare professionals who honor your viewpoints and help you to obtain your goals.

Use the tools I've provided. Carefully examine your own health. We go around this life just one time, but many of us live as if we have 500 years. Often times, people focus too much on the *quantity* of life—how many years they can live, according to their family genetics and statistics. I would like to live as long as possible without sacrificing the *quality*. I want to be able to enjoy my life with my family and friends by doing all of the things that make me happy both at work and at play. After all, what's the point of being one hundred years old and morbid?

Share this knowledge with your family and friends. Let's help change the world. The decisions that you make, starting right now, can make the difference you deserve!